TABLE OF CONTENTS

INTRODUCTION

Obesity is reaching epidemic proportions in Western countries and is a strong risk factor for cardiovascular disease. Despite health care organizations constantly recommend to control the weight, this goal often fails. It is well known that exercise and diet are two key factors for the control of body weight, but the ideal amount and type of exercise and also the ideal diet for weight control are still under debate. A widely accepted nutritional regime is the Mediterranean diet that provides evident health benefits; however, these effects may be due to other lifestyle factors which may contribute to the health benefits perhaps as much as specific food choices. There are several other options available to produce good weight loss results, also for maintenance of the goal achieved. One of these strategies is the VLCKD (very low calorie ketogenic diet). This diet has a solid physiological and biochemical basis which is able to induce effective weight loss and improvement of several parameters of cardiovascular risk.

In this e-book, I present my personalized version of VLCKD, with an example of meal plan and some indication to maintain the weight loss achieved. I also describe my personal experience with VLCKD, hoping that my contribution can be somehow useful to everyone who wants to undertake this diet and adopt an healthier lifestyle.

ABOUT ME

I got my M.Sc. in Industrial Biotechnology in 2012 (University of Milano Bicocca, Italy), then I became qualified as Professional Biologist in 2013 (University of Insubria, Italy) and I took my PhD in Life Sciences in 2016 (University of Milano Bicocca, Italy, and KU Leuven, Belgium). Now I work as Biologist Nutritionist in my own studio "GDS Nutrizione" (www.gdsnutrizione.it), located in Northern Italy.

Very Low Calorie Ketogenic Diet (VLCKD)

- Mediterranean Style -

What is a VLCKD? And why to choose it?

This diet is useful when we want to lose body fat, as the caloric intake is very low (about **800 kcal** per day) but the protein intake is high enough to maintaint muscle mass. By contrast, carbohydrates and fats are strongly reduced, so that our body must use storage fat as energy source, in a process called **β**-oxidation.

The final products of this metabolic pathway are **ketone bodies**, which can suppress hunger: thus, we will be able to follow this strict diet without suffering.

VLCKD allows to reach the desired weight in a shorter time than traditional hypocaloric diets (about 1-1.5 kg per week, depending on sex, body mass and exercise) without reducing muscle mass. Indeed, **muscle mass is preserved** by an adequate protein intake, which is tailored to every person. Talking about protein, this is not a hyperproteic diet; instead, it is a normoproteic diet, with high biological value protein.

As proteins are enough to sustain muscle mass, **weight loss is almost totally at the expense of fats**; additionally, the satiating effect of proteins and the presence of ketone bodies derived from the use of storage fats help to **suppress hunger** (always present in traditional hypocaloric diets) starting from the 2nd-3rd day of VLCKD.

During a VLCKD, however, carbohydrates are not completely excluded: 40-50 grams per day are able to avoid basal metabolism reduction, which could impair weight loss maintenance when VLCKD is completed.

Vitamin and mineral **supplementation** is necessary during VLCKD to avoid micronutrient deficiency.

Of course, VLCKD is a transition diet, that must be gradually followed by a healthy, balanced diet.

This is the reason why, at the end of VLCKD, dieters must transition off the ketogenic diet, for a time that is equal to the slimming phase. The **transition to a normal diet** is crucial and must be carefully applied, if we want to maintain the weight loss.

Why "Mediterranean"?

The Mediterranean diet is widely recognized as being one of the best diets for weight loss and overall health. When compared to a typical Western diet filled with processed foods, this plant-based diet is a safe, effective, and reliable choice.

On the other hand, the ketogenic diet has a greater potential to make significant changes on several conditions ranging from diabetes and obesity to neurological disorders like Alzheimer's disease, Parkinson's disease, and epilepsy.

Therefore, the Mediterranean diet and the ketogenic diet both have significant advantages under different contexts. When we combine them into one diet, most of their downsides melt away, providing us with a way of eating that can significantly improve every aspect of health.

A **ketogenic Mediterranean diet** incorporates extra virgin olive oil as the principal source of fat, green vegetables and salads as the main source of carbohydrates, and fish as the main source of protein. Moreover, since legumes are another food that is very present in the Mediterranean diet but contain a moderate quantity of carbohydrates, I decided to add low-carb soy products, like tofu and tempeh, to my Mediterranean VLCKD. The process of making tofu is relatively similar to the way that cheese is made from milk, while tempeh is fermented: fermentation removes most of the carbohydrates, leaving us the possibility to add a source of vegetable protein to our ketogenic diet. Tempeh is known to reduce cholesterol, increase bone density, reduce menopausal symptoms and promote muscle recovery. In addition to these amazing benefits, tempeh has the same protein quality as meat and contains high levels of vitamins B5, B6, B3 and B2.

VLCKD steps

In the first step, which has a duration of **21 days**, only lean proteins (meat, fish, eggs) and low-carbohydrate vegetables are eaten, with a low intake of dressing oil. During this phase, ketosis is reached, so that the dieters don't feel hungry and storage fats are used to produce energy.

In the second step, called **transition phase**, dieters will gradually increase carbohydrate amount (fruits, bread, rice, etc.) until they reach a normal and balanced diet. Only if they exercise, they will lose extra weight during this phase; otherwise, they'll have a weight stabilisation, which CANNOT be reached if they won't follow this meal plan.

When VLCKD is NOT recommended

- ✓ Kidney failure (if serum creatinine is more than 1.5 mg/dl, normal protein intake must be reduced)
- ✓ Acute liver failure (fatty acid oxidation occurs in the liver)
- ✓ Type-1 diabetes (ketoacidosis occurs)
- ✓ Heart failure (wrong use of sodium)
- ✓ Pregnancy and breastfeeding
- ✓ Severe mental disorders
- ✓ Growing children.

which are the foods that I can eat during VLCKD?

The choice of allowed foods is pretty limited. You can combine one of the food items in each following categories, to obtain a meal composed by protein + vegetables + oil:

PROTEIN SOURCES

- ✓ Lean meat (skinless chicken and turkey, horse, lamb, cattle steaks, pork chops with the fat trimmed off, burgers and meatballs from lean meat, lean cured meat such as bresaola or low-in-fat ham)
- ✓ Fish (sea fish, river fish or lake fish)
- ✓ Eggs (limiting egg yolk, as it is rich in fats, and preferring egg white)
- ✓ Vegan sources as tofu or tempeh (it is always important to verify that carbohydrate amount is low, as it may vary between different products)

VEGETABLES

Prefer low-carbohydrate vegetables, such as:

- ✓ Cucumbers
- ✓ Iceberg lettuce
- ✓ Celery
- ✓ White mushrooms
- ✓ Spinach
- ✓ Swiss chard

- ✓ Broccoli
- ✓ Bell peppers
- ✓ Zucchini
- ✓ Cauliflower
- ✓ Asparagus
- ✓ Alfalfa sprouts
- ✓ Radishes
- ✓ Arugula
- ✓ Radicchio
- ✓ Tomatoes
- ✓ Fermented vegetables (which contain gut healthy probiotics; check the list of ingredients to make sure no sugar was added)

DRESSING OILS

- ✓ Extra virgin olive oil
- ✓ Extra virgin unrefined coconut oil
- ✓ Organic and grass fed butter/ghee

FREELY CONSUMABLE FOODS: sugar-free drinks, coffee and tea, vinegar, pepper, onion, garlic, spices, herbs such as origan or basil.

FOOD SUPPLEMENTS: sugar-free potassium + magnesium, multivitamin/multimineral, probiotics, sugar-free psyllium husk powder (if stipsis occurs).

21-DAY MEAL PLAN

DAY 1

Breakfast	Tea or coffee with sweetener + Optional: 50-100 ml skimmed milk + 30 g isolated lean whey protein, dissolved in water + Magnesium and potassium + Probiotics + Multivitamin/multimineral
Lunch	150 g tofu with 3-4 dried tomatoes and 3-4 anchovies in olive oil + 200 g vegetable soup without potatoes and legumes (cooked with a soup cube) + Optional: coffee with sweetener
Dinner	200 g trout (cooked with salt, pepper, Herbes de Provence and white wine) + 200 g Radicchio (Italian chicory) and tomatoes (dressed with 10 g extra virgin olive oil and vinegar) + Herbal tea + 10 g extra dark chocolate 90-95% cocoa

If you feel hungry during the day, drink tea or herbal tea and eat raw fibrous vegetables such as fennels or celeri.

Drink at least 2 litres of water, including tea and herbal tea.

DAY 2

Breakfast	Tea or coffee with sweetener + Optional: 50-100 ml skimmed milk + 30 g isolated lean whey protein, dissolved in water + Magnesium and potassium + Probiotics + Multivitamin/multimineral
Lunch	250 g chicken breast (cooked with salt, pepper, Herbes de Provence, white wine) + 200 g Radicchio (Italian chicory) and tomatoes (dressed with 10 g extra virgin olive oil and vinegar) + Optional: coffee with sweetener
Dinner	150 g egg white + 1 whole egg (cooked with 5 g extra virgin olive oil, salt, pepper, onion) + 200 g cubed pumpkin (cooked with 5 g extra virgin olive oil, white wine, a soup cube, rosemary) + Herbal tea + 10 g extra dark chocolate 90-95% cocoa

If you feel hungry during the day, drink tea or herbal tea and eat raw fibrous vegetables such as fennels or celeri.

Drink at least 2 litres of water, including tea and herbal tea.

DAY 3

Breakfast	Tea or coffee with sweetener + Optional: 50-100 ml skimmed milk + 30 g isolated lean whey protein, dissolved in water + Magnesium and potassium + Probiotics + Multivitamin/multimineral
Lunch	100 g wild smoked salmon + 200 g spinach (cooked with 10 g organic butter) + Optional: coffee with sweetener
Dinner	Omelet made with: 150 g egg white + 1 whole egg + 10 g organic butter or extra virgin olive oil + salt + pepper + 200 g sliced zucchini + Herbal tea + 10 g extra dark chocolate 90-95% cocoa

If you feel hungry during the day, drink tea or herbal tea and eat raw fibrous vegetables such as fennels or celeri.

Drink at least 2 litres of water, including tea and herbal tea.

DAY 4

Breakfast	Tea or coffee with sweetener + Optional: 50-100 ml skimmed milk + 30 g isolated lean whey protein, dissolved in water + Magnesium and potassium + Probiotics + Multivitamin/multimineral
Lunch	100 g lean ham + 200 g cauliflower (boiled in salty hot water and then dressed with 10 g extra virgin olive oil) + Optional: coffee with sweetener
Dinner	150 g tunafish (cooked with 5 g extra virgin olive oil, origan, salt, pepper) + 200 g asparagus (boiled in salty hot water and then dressed with 5 g extra virgin olive oil) + Herbal tea + 10 g extra dark chocolate 90-95% cocoa

If you feel hungry during the day, drink tea or herbal tea and eat raw fibrous vegetables such as fennels or celeri.

Drink at least 2 litres of water, including tea and herbal tea.

DAY 5

Breakfast	Tea or coffee with sweetener + Optional: 50-100 ml skimmed milk + 30 g isolated lean whey protein, dissolved in water + Magnesium and potassium + Probiotics + Multivitamin/multimineral
Lunch	250 g codfish (cooked with cherry tomatoes, basil, salt, pepper and 5 g extra virgin olive oil) + 200 g vegetable soup without potatoes and legumes (cooked with a soup cube) + Optional: coffee with sweetener
Dinner	150 g escalope of veal (cooked with 5 g extra virgin olive oil, origan, salt, tomato sauce) + 200 g broccoli (boiled in salty hot water and then dressed with 5 g extra virgin olive oil) + Herbal tea + 10 g extra dark chocolate 90-95% cocoa

If you feel hungry during the day, drink tea or herbal tea and eat raw fibrous vegetables such as fennels or celeri.

Drink at least 2 litres of water, including tea and herbal tea.

DAY 6

Breakfast	Tea or coffee with sweetener + Optional: 50-100 ml skimmed milk + 30 g isolated lean whey protein, dissolved in water + Magnesium and potassium + Probiotics + Multivitamin/multimineral
Lunch	150 g tempeh with tomato sauce, basil, salt, pepper and 5 g extra virgin olive oil + 200 g white mushrooms (cooked with half soup cube, white wine, parsley and 5 g extra virgin olive oil) + Optional: coffee with sweetener
Dinner	Omelet made with: 150 g egg white + 1 whole egg + 10 g organic butter or extra virgin coconut oil + salt + pepper + onion + 200 g asparagus + Herbal tea + 10 g extra dark chocolate 90-95% cocoa

If you feel hungry during the day, drink tea or herbal tea and eat raw fibrous vegetables such as fennels or celeri.

Drink at least 2 litres of water, including tea and herbal tea.

DAY 7

Breakfast	Tea or coffee with sweetener + Optional: 50-100 ml skimmed milk + 30 g isolated lean whey protein, dissolved in water + Magnesium and potassium + Probiotics + Multivitamin/multimineral
Lunch	250 g grilled cuttlefish with salt, pepper and 5 g extra virgin olive oil + 200 g thinly-sliced fennel with salt, pepper, vinegar, 5 g extra virgin olive oil + Optional: coffee with sweetener
Dinner	100 g grilled turkey hamburger + 200 g mixed vegetables (zucchini, eggplant, peppers, onion, cooked with half soup cube and 10 g extra virgin olive oil) + Herbal tea + 10 g extra dark chocolate 90-95% cocoa

If you feel hungry during the day, drink tea or herbal tea and eat raw fibrous vegetables such as fennels or celeri.

Drink at least 2 litres of water, including tea and herbal tea.

DAY 8

Breakfast	Tea or coffee with sweetener + Optional: 50-100 ml skimmed milk + 30 g isolated lean whey protein, dissolved in water + Magnesium and potassium + Probiotics + Multivitamin/multimineral
Lunch	150 g tofu with cherry tomatoes, basil, salt, pepper and 5 g extra virgin olive oil + 200 g Brussels sprouts (steamed and then dressed with 5 g extra virgin olive oil) + Optional: coffee with sweetener
Dinner	150 g grilled pork steak (with salt and pepper) + 200 g mixed vegetables (zucchini, eggplant, peppers, onion, cooked with half soup cube and 10 g extra virgin olive oil) + Herbal tea + 10 g extra dark chocolate 90-95% cocoa

If you feel hungry during the day, drink tea or herbal tea and eat raw fibrous vegetables such as fennels or celeri.

Drink at least 2 litres of water, including tea and herbal tea.

DAY 9

Breakfast	Tea or coffee with sweetener + Optional: 50-100 ml skimmed milk + 30 g isolated lean whey protein, dissolved in water + Magnesium and potassium + Probiotics + Multivitamin/multimineral
Lunch	250 g grilled shrimps with salt and pepper + 200 g cubed pumpkin (cooked with 10 g extra virgin olive oil, white wine, a soup cube, rosemary) + Optional: coffee with sweetener
Dinner	100 g lean ham (or Bresaola or Prosciutto) + 200 g zucchini cream (combine chicken broth, 10 g extra virgin olive oil, onion, pepper, garlic and zucchini in a large pot over medium heat and bring to a boil. Cook for about 20 minutes, then purée with an immersion blender) + Herbal tea + 10 g extra dark chocolate 90-95% cocoa

If you feel hungry during the day, drink tea or herbal tea and eat raw fibrous vegetables such as fennels or celeri.

Drink at least 2 litres of water, including tea and herbal tea.

DAY 10

Breakfast	Tea or coffee with sweetener + Optional: 50-100 ml skimmed milk + 30 g isolated lean whey protein, dissolved in water + Magnesium and potassium + Probiotics + Multivitamin/multimineral
Lunch	150 g grilled tempeh with salt, pepper, basil and 5 g extra virgin olive oil + 200 g broccoli (steamed and then dressed with 5 g extra virgin olive oil) + Optional: coffee with sweetener
Dinner	150 g grilled veal fillet (with salt, pepper) + 200 g leek and spinach soup (combine chicken broth, 10 g extra virgin olive oil, onion, pepper, garlic, leek and spinach in a large pot over medium heat and bring to a boil. Cook for about 20 minutes, then purée with an immersion blender) + Herbal tea + 10 g extra dark chocolate 90-95% cocoa

If you feel hungry during the day, drink tea or herbal tea and eat raw fibrous vegetables such as fennels or celeri.

Drink at least 2 litres of water, including tea and herbal tea.

DAY 11

Breakfast	Tea or coffee with sweetener + Optional: 50-100 ml skimmed milk + 30 g isolated lean whey protein, dissolved in water + Magnesium and potassium + Probiotics + Multivitamin/multimineral
Lunch	150 g grilled tunafish with salt, pepper, Herbes de Provence (then add 5 g extra virgin olive oil) + 200 g lettuce, cherry tomatoes, radishes (dressed with vinegar and 5 g extra virgin olive oil) + Optional: coffee with sweetener
Dinner	Omelet made with: 150 g egg white + 1 whole egg + 10 g organic butter or extra virgin olive oil + salt + pepper + 200 g sliced zucchini + Herbal tea + 10 g extra dark chocolate 90-95% cocoa

If you feel hungry during the day, drink tea or herbal tea and eat raw fibrous vegetables such as fennels or celeri.

Drink at least 2 litres of water, including tea and herbal tea.

DAY 12

Breakfast	Tea or coffee with sweetener + Optional: 50-100 ml skimmed milk + 30 g isolated lean whey protein, dissolved in water + Magnesium and potassium + Probiotics + Multivitamin/multimineral
Lunch	150 g tofu with tomato sauce, 3 green olives, salt, pepper and 5 g extra virgin olive oil + 200 g white mushrooms (cooked with half soup cube, white wine, parsley and 5 g extra virgin olive oil) + Optional: coffee with sweetener
Dinner	200 g roast beef (cold or hot) + 200 g cauliflower (boiled in salty hot water and then dressed with 10 g extra virgin olive oil) + Herbal tea + 10 g extra dark chocolate 90-95% cocoa

If you feel hungry during the day, drink tea or herbal tea and eat raw fibrous vegetables such as fennels or celeri.

Drink at least 2 litres of water, including tea and herbal tea.

DAY 13

Breakfast	Tea or coffee with sweetener + Optional: 50-100 ml skimmed milk + 30 g isolated lean whey protein, dissolved in water + Magnesium and potassium + Probiotics + Multivitamin/multimineral
Lunch	100 g wild smoked salmon + 200 g cucumbers, celeri, tomatoes and arugula salad (dressed with vinegar and 10 g extra virgin olive oil) + Optional: coffee with sweetener
Dinner	100 g grilled chicken hamburger (add rosemary, salt and pepper) + 200 g mixed vegetables (zucchini, carrots, asparagus, onion, cooked with half soup cube and 10 g extra virgin olive oil) + Herbal tea + 10 g extra dark chocolate 90-95% cocoa

If you feel hungry during the day, drink tea or herbal tea and eat raw fibrous vegetables such as fennels or celeri.

Drink at least 2 litres of water, including tea and herbal tea.

DAY 14

Breakfast	Tea or coffee with sweetener + Optional: 50-100 ml skimmed milk + 30 g isolated lean whey protein, dissolved in water + Magnesium and potassium + Probiotics + Multivitamin/multimineral
Lunch	250 g stone bass fillet (cooked with tomato sauce, basil, 3-4 green olives, salt, pepper and 10 g extra virgin olive oil) + 200 g vegetable soup without potatoes and legumes (cooked with a soup cube) + Optional: coffee with sweetener
Dinner	Omelet made with: 150 g egg white + 1 whole egg + 10 g organic butter or extra virgin coconut oil + salt + pepper + onion + 200 g asparagus + Herbal tea + 10 g extra dark chocolate 90-95% cocoa

If you feel hungry during the day, drink tea or herbal tea and eat raw fibrous vegetables such as fennels or celeri.

Drink at least 2 litres of water, including tea and herbal tea.

DAY 15

Breakfast	Tea or coffee with sweetener + Optional: 50-100 ml skimmed milk + 30 g isolated lean whey protein, dissolved in water + Magnesium and potassium + Probiotics + Multivitamin/multimineral
Lunch	200 g grilled chicken breast (add salt, pepper and sage) + 200 g spinach (cooked with 10 g organic butter) + Optional: coffee with sweetener
Dinner	150 g grilled tempeh with salt, pepper, rosemary and 5 g extra virgin olive oil + 200 g broccoli (steamed and then dressed with 5 g extra virgin olive oil) + Herbal tea + 10 g extra dark chocolate 90-95% cocoa

If you feel hungry during the day, drink tea or herbal tea and eat raw fibrous vegetables such as fennels or celeri.

Drink at least 2 litres of water, including tea and herbal tea.

DAY 16

Breakfast	Tea or coffee with sweetener + Optional: 50-100 ml skimmed milk + 30 g isolated lean whey protein, dissolved in water + Magnesium and potassium + Probiotics + Multivitamin/multimineral
Lunch	150 g tunafish (cooked with 5 g extra virgin olive oil, origan, salt, pepper) + 200 g asparagus (boiled in salty hot water and then dressed with 5 g extra virgin olive oil) + Optional: coffee with sweetener
Dinner	150 g grilled pork steak (+ salt, pepper) + 200 g mixed vegetables (zucchini, eggplant, peppers, onion, cooked with half soup cube and 10 g extra virgin olive oil) + Herbal tea + 10 g extra dark chocolate 90-95% cocoa

If you feel hungry during the day, drink tea or herbal tea and eat raw fibrous vegetables such as fennels or celeri.

Drink at least 2 litres of water, including tea and herbal tea.

DAY 17

Breakfast	Tea or coffee with sweetener + Optional: 50-100 ml skimmed milk + 30 g isolated lean whey protein, dissolved in water + Magnesium and potassium + Probiotics + Multivitamin/multimineral
Lunch	150 g egg white + 1 whole egg (cooked with 5 g extra virgin olive oil, salt, pepper, onion) + 200 g cubed pumpkin (cooked with 5 g extra virgin olive oil, white wine, a soup cube, sage and origan) + Optional: coffee with sweetener
Dinner	100 g grilled turkey hamburger + 200 g cauliflower soup (combine chicken broth, 10 g olive oil, onion, pepper and cauliflower in a pot over medium heat and bring to a boil. Cook for about 20 minutes, then purée with an immersion blender) + Herbal tea + 10 g extra dark chocolate 90-95% cocoa

If you feel hungry during the day, drink tea or herbal tea and eat raw fibrous vegetables such as fennels or celeri.

Drink at least 2 litres of water, including tea and herbal tea.

DAY 18

Breakfast	Tea or coffee with sweetener + Optional: 50-100 ml skimmed milk + 30 g isolated lean whey protein, dissolved in water + Magnesium and potassium + Probiotics + Multivitamin/multimineral
Lunch	100 g lean ham (or Bresaola or Prosciutto) + 200 g Iceberg lettuce and tomatoes (dressed with 10 g extra virgin olive oil and vinegar) + Optional: coffee with sweetener
Dinner	200 g trout (cooked with salt, pepper, Herbes de Provence and white wine) + 200 g stewed fennel (dressed with 10 g olive oil, salt, parsley and pepper) + Herbal tea + 10 g extra dark chocolate 90-95% cocoa

If you feel hungry during the day, drink tea or herbal tea and eat raw fibrous vegetables such as fennels or celeri.

Drink at least 2 litres of water, including tea and herbal tea.

DAY 19

Breakfast	Tea or coffee with sweetener + Optional: 50-100 ml skimmed milk + 30 g isolated lean whey protein, dissolved in water + Magnesium and potassium + Probiotics + Multivitamin/multimineral
Lunch	150 g grilled veal fillet (with salt, pepper) + 200 g Brussels sprouts (steamed and then dressed with 5 g extra virgin olive oil) + Optional: coffee with sweetener
Dinner	200 g cubed perch fillet (cooked with cherry tomatoes, parsley, garlic, salt, pepper and 10 g extra virgin olive oil) + 200 g vegetable soup without potatoes and legumes (cooked with a soup cube) + Herbal tea + 10 g extra dark chocolate 90-95% cocoa

If you feel hungry during the day, drink tea or herbal tea and eat raw fibrous vegetables such as fennels or celeri.

Drink at least 2 litres of water, including tea and herbal tea.

DAY 20

Breakfast	Tea or coffee with sweetener + Optional: 50-100 ml skimmed milk + 30 g isolated lean whey protein, dissolved in water + Magnesium and potassium + Probiotics + Multivitamin/multimineral
Lunch	150 g tofu with 3-4 dried tomatoes and 3-4 anchovies in olive oil + 200 g white mushrooms (cooked with half soup cube, white wine, parsley and 5 g extra virgin olive oil) + Optional: coffee with sweetener
Dinner	Omelet made with: 150 g egg white + 1 whole egg + 10 g organic butter or extra virgin coconut oil + salt + pepper + onion + 200 g asparagus + Herbal tea + 10 g extra dark chocolate 90-95% cocoa

If you feel hungry during the day, drink tea or herbal tea and eat raw fibrous vegetables such as fennels or celeri.

Drink at least 2 litres of water, including tea and herbal tea.

DAY 21

Breakfast	Tea or coffee with sweetener + Optional: 50-100 ml skimmed milk + 30 g isolated lean whey protein, dissolved in water + Magnesium and potassium + Probiotics + Multivitamin/multimineral
Lunch	150 g escalope of veal (cooked with 5 g extra virgin olive oil, origan, salt, tomato sauce) + 200 g mixed vegetables (zucchini, carrots, onion, cooked with half soup cube and 10 g extra virgin olive oil) + Optional: coffee with sweetener
Dinner	100 g wild smoked salmon + 200 g cucumbers, celeri, tomatoes and arugula salad (dressed with vinegar and 10 g extra virgin olive oil) + Herbal tea + 10 g extra dark chocolate 90-95% cocoa

If you feel hungry during the day, drink tea or herbal tea and eat raw fibrous vegetables such as fennels or celeri.

Drink at least 2 litres of water, including tea and herbal tea.

AND NOW...THE TRANSITION PHASE

Now that you finished with your 21 days of VLCKD, you can start with the second step, the **transition phase**, so that you will **gradually** increase carbohydrate amount (fruits, bread, rice, etc.) until you reach a normal and balanced diet. Why gradually? Because in the VLCKD you eat less than 30 g of carbohydrate, that slightly stimulate insulin secretion; thus, your body has to get used to secrete the correct amount of insulin again. Moreover, during the VLCKD you eat few calories (about 800 kcal), so metabolism has to boost when you increase your caloric intake during the transition phase.

To ensure weight fixation during the transition phase, regular exercise is strongly recommended.

The transition phase has the same duration as the VLCKD (i.e. 21 days) and is further divided into three steps, that you should follow carefully in order to avoid a weight gain once VLCKD is finished.

Here are the three steps:

STEP 1 – WEEK 1 OF THE TRANSITION PHASE (DAYS 22 TO 28 IF YOU COUNT FROM THE FIRST DAY OF VLCKD)

In this first phase, you can add **fruit** to your VLCKD in two moments of the day. If you prefer to have a break, you can eat 150 g of fruit (no matter the type) between breakfast and lunch and 150 g of fruit between lunch and dinner. Otherwise, you can eat your fruits at the end of your lunch and dinner. Usually this option is better, since you won't stimulate insulin secretion as you would do by eating your fruits isolated (other nutrients of the meal -such as protein, fat and fiber- will help to lower glycemic load).

In addition to fruit, you can eat a pot (150-170 g) of sugar-free **white Greek yogurt**, that you can enrich with some nuts, erythritol/stevia, sugar-free cocoa powder and small pieces of extra dark chocolate. Feel free to choose the best moment of the day to enjoy your Greek yogurt.

If you prefer to taste a salty dairy product instead of a Greek yogurt, you can eat 100-150 g of a **fresh cheese**, like ricotta, creamy goat cheese, mozzarella, feta, cottage cheese or quark.

STEP 2 – WEEK 2 OF THE TRANSITION PHASE (DAYS 29 TO 35 IF YOU COUNT FROM THE FIRST DAY OF VLCKD)

In the second step of the transition phase, you can also add **wholegrain bread** or **rye bread** to your daily meal plan: they are low-glycemic index (GI) bread types, so they won't stimulate insulin as white bread does. Another good choice may be **sourdough bread**, that has a lower GI due to the higher acidity level. Fibre, vitamin and mineral levels vary with the flour used, with wholegrain sourdough being the preferred choice. Be sure to choose an authentic sourdough, as some are faux sourdough and contain yeast rather than the traditional starter: authentic sourdough takes a long time to produce and results in an acidic and chewy bread, two features that lower the GI. Look for a chewy texture and the absence of yeast in the ingredients, preferably with wholewheat flour or rye wholemeal, grains and seeds.

Calculate about 60 grams of bread (i.e. two slices) that you can eat for lunch and for dinner.

STEP 3 – WEEK 3 OF THE TRANSITION PHASE (DAYS 36 TO 42 IF YOU COUNT FROM THE FIRST DAY OF VLCKD)

In the final part of the transition phase, you can re-introduce **wholegrain cereals and pseudocereals** such as wheat, rice, barley, maize, rye, oats, millets, sorghum, amaranth, buckwheat, quinoa. Otherwise, you can re-introduce **legumes**, such as alfalfa, beans, peas, chickpeas, lentils, lupins, soybeans. Third option: you can alternate cereals and legumes during Week 3. The right serving size is 60 grams of cereals (to weight uncooked) and of 50 grams of legumes (if dry and uncooked; otherwise, 150 grams of cooked legumes).

During the transition phase, you may **continue to lose weight**, as caloric intake is still lower than basal metabolic rate until you reach a normocaloric, balanced diet. By contrast, many people increase their weight of about 1-2 kilos during carbohydrate re-introduction: don't panic, it's not fat, it's only the water attached to carbohydrates!

When you re-introduce carbohydrates, your body will stop to produce and to use ketone bodies, that usually help to reduce hunger, so it is normal during the transition phase that **you feel more hungry** than during the VLCKD even though you eat more calories. You have to be patient and use tricks to avoid to fall into temptation, like drinking, eating fibrous vegetables or simply get out of the kitchen and go outside for a walk (or a jog) and get your mind refocused on something besides food.

It is not always easy to properly follow the transition phase due to psychological problems: as you got back in shape, you might underestimate the importance of the transition phase and eat things that are not part of your prescribed diet (usually things like junk food). Nothing could be more wrong and dangerous! Indeed, your weight may go up again if you don't follow the transition phase in the right way.

After a good transition phase, the weight is well stabilized, but you cannot be sure that it won't go up again if you continue to follow a bad lifestyle. This is an unsolved problem with every type of diet: only if you adopt a **healthier lifestyle**, you can be pretty sure you won't regain weight.

Always try to study and understand what you are going to eat: only if you are aware of the food you incorporate in your diet, you will really and permanently change your life.

How to Behave After This Diet

Changing the way you eat can be easy. Start with small changes to make healthier choices you can enjoy. To start, learn about some of the worst food offenders (fast food, high-calorie desserts, sweet drinks, etc.) and how to replace them with healthier choices. Then try some portion-control tricks. The right mix can help you be healthier now and in the future: find your healthy eating style and maintain it for a lifetime.

Calorie-bomb food favorites

Most of daily calories in the Western diet come from foods high in fat and sugar. Sweets like cookies and cakes, along with yeast breads, are at the top of the list, as well as chicken dishes (often breaded and fried), sodas, and energy and sports drinks. Pizza, alcohol, pasta, tortilla dishes, and beef dishes pile on more calories.

Favorite foods like pizza may just need a makeover: pizza can have lots of calories, refined grains, and fats, but with a few tweaks, it can be OK once a week (or less!):

- ✔ Choose a thin, whole-grain crust.
- ✔ Pile on veggies and skip meat.
- ✔ Use low-fat or fat-free cheese or just a sprinkle.
- ✔ Have one small slice and fill the rest of your plate with vegetables.

To eat less

Just two problem foods (i.e. solid fats and added sugars) count for about 800 of daily calories. That's almost half the calories an average woman should have in a day. Cut calories by drinking water or unsweetened beverages; soda, energy drinks, and sports drinks are a major source of added sugars. Dietary guidelines say you should limit solid and saturated fats as while as rotally eliminate trans fat. Cut back on fast foods and refined grains, like white bread. While you're at it, cut down on sodium (salt) to avoid to raise your chances of high blood pressure and heart and kidney disease. Many processed foods contain high amounts of sodium. Choose fresh vegetables, meats, poultry, and seafood when possible. Using spices or herbs, such as dill, chili powder, paprika, or cumin, and lemon or lime juice, can add flavor without adding salt.

To eat more

Add more nutritious foods to your diet.

- ✓ Instead of fatty meats, choose lean protein and seafood. Eat at least 200 grams of fish 2-3 times per week. Vary your protein routine! For car trips, pack a mixture of unsalted nuts, seeds and dried fruit for a crunchy, protein-packed snack.
- ✓ Instead of solid fats like butter or margarine, use extra virgin olive oil, that is good for your waistline and heart.

What are solid fats? Fats that are solid at room temperature usually contain saturated and trans fats. Trans fats should be avoided as much as possible and saturated fats should only contribute 10% of your calories. You will find saturated fats in butter, coconut oil, animal fats in meat, dairy, bacon and chicken skin.

✓ Instead of baked goods and cereals with all white or refined grains, make at least half of your grains whole grains.

What are whole grains? The outer shell, or "bran," of a kernel of wheat, rice, barley, or other grain is full of fiber, vitamins, and minerals. Fiber helps you feel full on fewer calories and keeps your bathroom visits regular. But to make white (refined) flour from a kernel of wheat, food makers get rid of the bran: with it goes much of the fiber and vitamins.

✓ Other healthy choices: nonfat or low-fat dairy foods, eggs, beans, and lots of fruits and vegetables.
Make half your plate fruits and vegetables: focus on whole fruits and vary your veggies. Eat seasonally! Checking what fruits and vegetables are in season in your area can help save money. Craving something sweet? Try dried fruits like cranberries, mango, apricots, cherries, or raisins. To meet your fruit goal: keep fresh fruit rinsed and where you can see it. Reach for a piece when you need a snack.
Vary your veggies by adding a new vegetable to a different meal each day.

Add color to salads with baby carrots, shredded red cabbage, or green beans.

Vegetables go well with a dip or dressing. Try a low-fat dip or hummus with raw broccoli, red and yellow peppers, sugar snap peas, celery, cherry tomatoes or cauliflower.

Serving the right size

Start downsizing to healthy portions and your body will, too. Check food labels and restaurant menus for hidden calories. Learn to "eyeball" your food to assess what's too much and what's just right. Indeed, you don't need to weigh or measure your food every time you eat. Instead, keep a mental image of an object: this makes it easy for you imagine healthy portion sizes.

To shrink your portions:

- ✓ Eat from a smaller dish like a salad plate.
- ✓ Learn and serve the right-sized portion.
- ✓ Don't go back for seconds or keep extra food on the table to tempt you.
- ✓ Store leftovers in single-serving containers for quick meals.

Restaurants usually serve one person enough food for two or three, but you don't have to eat it all:

- ✓ Order a half portion or something from the kid's menu.
- ✓ If you order a full-size entree, box up half of it before you start eating.
- ✓ Split a dish with a friend.

✓ Eat a healthy appetizer and soup or salad instead of an entrée.

I think it is worth mentioning a useful tool, called **The Healthy Eating Plate** (created by nutrition experts at the Harvard T.H. Chan School of Public Health and editors at Harvard Health Publications), that provides detailed guidance, in a simple format, to help people make the best eating choices. Here it is:

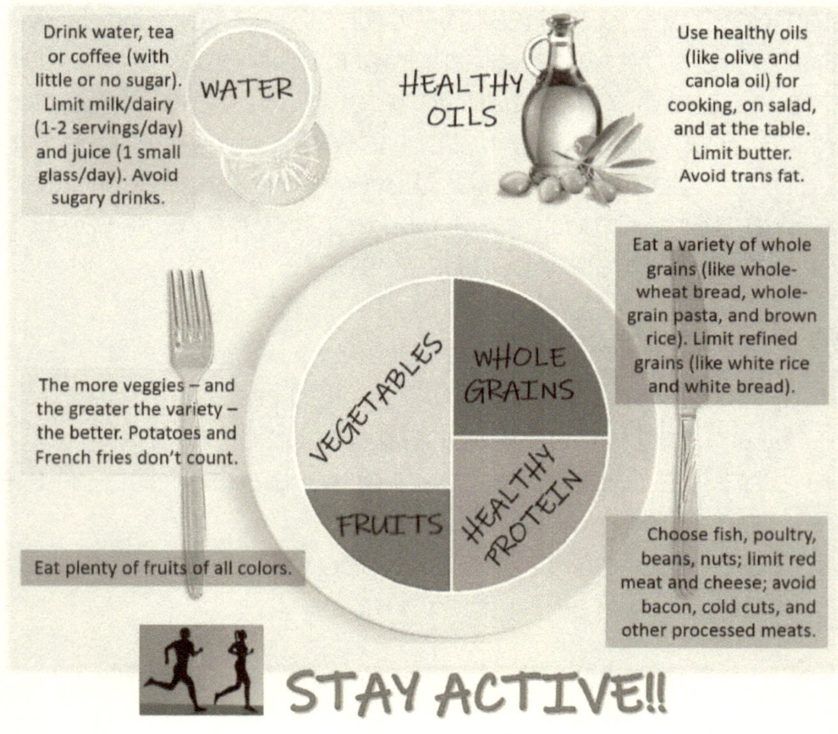

You can use the Healthy Eating Plate as a guide for creating healthy, balanced meals (whether served on a plate or packed in a lunch box). You can also put a copy on the fridge as a daily reminder to create healthy and balanced meals!

MY EXPERIENCE WITH VLCKD

Everybody I know could firmly say that I am addicted to sport, especially bike (road and mountain bike), running, skiing and mountain hiking. Everyday I need my "dose" of sport, otherwise I become nervous and I feel like I'm sick.

It is well known that sport performance increases if the percentage of storage body fat is limited (while essential body fat is necessary to maintain life and reproductive functions). For these reasons, I wanted to try the VLCKD to improve my body composition and lose a bit of fat, thus improving my athletic performances especially when I climb a mountain or a hill.

I chose this type of diet because I liked the fact that I could lose lots of kilos in few days, without sacrificing muscle mass and, above all, reducing exercise time and intensity only for 21 days. This latter point made me choose October and November to do my VLCKD, since this period is normally a "off-season": the ideal moment to improve body composition, thus starting a new sport season in the best possible way.

I was a little afraid of feeling always tired and hungry during the first 21 days, lacking energy to exercise. During the first three days, it was very difficult to me to eat only 800 kcal and skip snacks, as well as strongly reduce breakfast (my favorite daily meal). Considering my job, it was difficult to meet patients that talked about food every time, even more difficult to prepare them a meal plan.

Also, it was difficult to accept to reduce exercise duration and intensity (my legs couldn't work well without glycogen...). After this adaptation phase, I started feeling very well: the weight dropped quickly on the scale, I was active at work, the sleep improved, my intestine worked properly (while I often experience inflammation with "normal" nutrition), I felt like detoxified from carb craving and, to my great surprise, I felt light as a feather while I went running. Moreover, I didn't feel hungry (thanks to ketone bodies and protein), preparing my meals was very simple and quick and I started to eat slowly my food: that's a great thing to appreciate more what you're eating, to reach satiety and to avoid digestive problems.

I lost about 10% of my body weight during the first 21 days + transition phase, and my body fat percentage decreased from 22% to 17%. I continued to exercise every day also in the slimming phase, burning at least 400 kcal/day (and up to 600 kcal for some days).

I feel really satisfied after this period: a very short time to lose a lot of body fat, without affecting muscle mass and without suffering so much.

Now I'm ready to climb all mountains in the world! 

Gaia De Sanctis, PhD and Nutritionist

BIBLIOGRAPHY

Caprio M. et al. (2019) **Very-low-calorie ketogenic diet (VLCKD) in the management of metabolic diseases: systematic review and consensus statement from the Italian Society of Endocrinology (SIE)**. J Endocrinol Invest. 2019 Nov;42(11):1365-1386.

Tuttolomondo A. et al. (2019) **Metabolic and Vascular Effect of the Mediterranean Diet**. Int J Mol Sci. 2019 Sep 23;20(19).

Merra G. et al. (2017) **Effects of very-low-calorie diet on body composition, metabolic state, and genes expression: a randomized double-blind placebo-controlled trial**. Eur Rev Med Pharmacol Sci. 2017 Jan;21(2):329-345.

Castaldo G. et al. (2016) **An observational study of sequential protein-sparing, very low-calorie ketogenic diet (Oloproteic diet) and hypocaloric Mediterranean-like diet for the treatment of obesity**. Int J Food Sci Nutr. 2016 Sep;67(6):696-706.

Merra G. et al. (2016) **Very-low-calorie ketogenic diet with aminoacid supplement versus very low restricted-calorie diet for preserving muscle mass during weight loss: a pilot double-blind study**. Eur Rev Med Pharmacol Sci. 2016 Jul;20(12):2613-21.

Paoli A. et al. (2015) **Ketosis, ketogenic diet and food intake control: a complex relationship**. Front Psychol. 2015 Feb 2;6:27.

Paoli A. et al. (2013) **Long term successful weight loss with a combination biphasic ketogenic Mediterranean diet and Mediterranean diet maintenance protocol**. Nutrients. 2013 Dec 18;5(12):5205-17.

Bueno NB. et al. (2013) **Very-low-carbohydrate ketogenic diet v. low-fat diet for long-term weight loss: a meta-analysis of randomised controlled trials**. Br J Nutr. 2013 Oct;110(7):1178-87.

Paoli A. et al. (2011) **The ketogenic diet: an underappreciated therapeutic option?**. Clin Ter. 2011;162(5):e145-53.

Paoli A. et al. (2011) **Effect of ketogenic Mediterranean diet with phytoextracts and low carbohydrates/high-protein meals on weight, cardiovascular risk factors, body composition and diet compliance in Italian council employees**. Nutr J. 2011 Oct 12;10:112.

Adam-Perrot A. et al. (2006) **Low-carbohydrate diets: nutritional and physiological aspects**. Obes Rev. 2006 Feb;7(1):49-58.

Volek JS, Sharman MJ. (2004) **Cardiovascular and hormonal aspects of very-low-carbohydrate ketogenic diets**. Obes Res. 2004 Nov;12 Suppl 2:115S-23S.

Lyle McDonald (1998) **The Ketogenic Diet: a Complete Guide for the Dieter and the Practitioner**. ISBN 0-9671456-0-0.

Atkinson RL, Kaiser DL. (1985) **Effects of calorie restriction and weight loss on glucose and insulin levels in obese humans**. J Am Coll Nutr. 1985;4(4):411-9.

Harvard T.H. Chan – School of Public Health - "Healthy Eating Plate": https://www.hsph.harvard.edu/nutritionsource/healthy-eating-plate/